Lite'n Up

LAUGH YOURSELF

Skinny

Lite'n Up
LAUGH YOURSELF
Skinny

SAMARA Q. KLEIN

plain white **press**™

WHITE PLAINS, NY

First Edition, 2009

Published in the United States by Plain White Press
09 10 11 12 13 10 9 8 7 6 5 4 3 2 1

Library of Congress Control Number: 2008941461

ISBN 978-0-9777383-5-9

Book and cover design by Empire Design Studio
Illustration by Helen Dardik

This book is printed in China

Discover more at www.plainwhitepress.com and www.samaralitenup.com

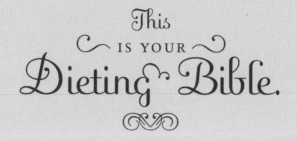

This
— IS YOUR —
Dieting Bible.

HOW IT Works

» Get up.

» Record the date.

» Step on the scale.

» Record your weight.

» Read today's funny reminder.

» Eat. (not much)

» Write down what you eat. (notice there's not much space)

» Overcome temptation. (see funny reminder)

» Write down your dieting hits and bombs.

By the time you fill this notebook, you'll be slim –
it's so easy, it's funny.

Chart of (vertical) pounds lost over weeks

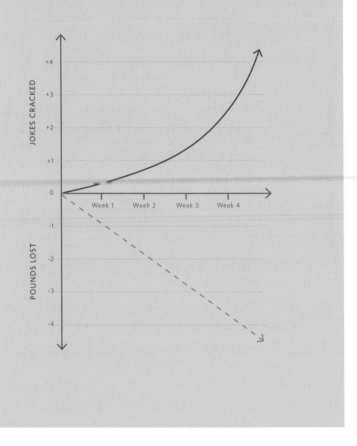

date & **WEIGHT**	/ /	

BREAKFAST

LUNCH

DINNER

FRUIT N' VEG	① ② ③ ④ ⑤ ⑥ ⑦
WATER	① ② ③ ④ ⑤ ⑥ ⑦

hits & **BOMBS**

date & **WEIGHT**	...... / ...... / ......
BREAKFAST	
LUNCH	
DINNER	
FRUIT N' VEG	① ② ③ ④ ⑤ ⑥ ⑦
WATER	① ② ③ ④ ⑤ ⑥ ⑦
hits & **BOMBS**	

IF YOU HAD TO CHOOSE,
WHICH WOULD YOU TAKE?

a) great sex

b) fettuccine alfredo

HELPFUL THOUGHT: you *do* have to choose.

If you eat something,
but no one else sees you eat it,
it has no calories.

And if you believe that,

let me tell you about the fail-safe
Chocolate Weight-Loss Diet.

date & **WEIGHT**	.........../.........../...........

BREAKFAST

LUNCH

DINNER

FRUIT N' VEG	① ② ③ ④ ⑤ ⑥ ⑦
WATER	① ② ③ ④ ⑤ ⑥ ⑦

hits & **BOMBS**

date & **WEIGHT**	....../....../......	
BREAKFAST		
LUNCH		
DINNER		
FRUIT N' VEG	① ② ③ ④ ⑤ ⑥ ⑦	
WATER	① ② ③ ④ ⑤ ⑥ ⑦	
hits & **BOMBS**		

On Mars,

a 180-pound person only weighs 68 pounds.

It takes a few months to get there,
so bring a snack.

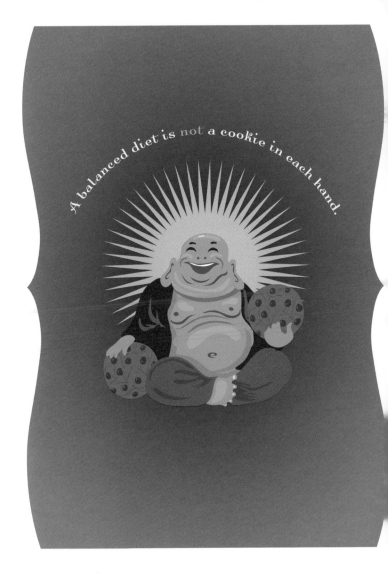

∂ate & **WEIGHT**	......../......../........
BREAKFAST	
LUNCH	
DINNER	
FRUIT N' VEG	① ② ③ ④ ⑤ ⑥ ⑦
WATER	① ② ③ ④ ⑤ ⑥ ⑦
hits & **BOMBS**	

date &
WEIGHT

.... / .... / ....

BREAKFAST

LUNCH

DINNER

FRUIT N' VEG ① ② ③ ④ ⑤ ⑥ ⑦

WATER ① ② ③ ④ ⑤ ⑥ ⑦

hits &
BOMBS

Samara Says

Inside every thin person is a fat person
waiting to get out and **ruin** your life.

Eat a peach,

but skip the
peach pound cake.

In other words, be ounce-wise, but **not** pound-cake-foolish.

date & **WEIGHT**	.... / .... /	
BREAKFAST		
LUNCH		
DINNER		
FRUIT N' VEG	① ② ③ ④ ⑤ ⑥ ⑦	
WATER	① ② ③ ④ ⑤ ⑥ ⑦	
hits & **BOMBS**		

| date &
WEIGHT | ..../......./............ | |

BREAKFAST

LUNCH

DINNER

| **FRUIT N' VEG** | ① ② ③ ④ ⑤ ⑥ ⑦ |
| **WATER** | ① ② ③ ④ ⑤ ⑥ ⑦ |

hits &
BOMBS

FOOD FOR THOUGHT:

Thoughts of food are **calorie-free**. Hold that thought and your **mouth closed**.

If you eat **5** cookies a day for a year that's **1,825** cookies.

If each of those cookies is **5** grams of fat, that's **9,125** grams of fat.

You don't need to be a mathematician to draw some serious conclusions from that.

date & WEIGHT	...... / ...... /	

BREAKFAST

LUNCH

DINNER

FRUIT N' VEG	① ② ③ ④ ⑤ ⑥ ⑦
WATER	① ② ③ ④ ⑤ ⑥ ⑦

hits & BOMBS

date & **WEIGHT**	......../......../........	
BREAKFAST	
LUNCH	
DINNER	
FRUIT N' VEG	① ② ③ ④ ⑤ ⑥ ⑦
WATER	① ② ③ ④ ⑤ ⑥ ⑦
hits & **BOMBS**	

Visualization exercise:
Picture a double chocolate fudge sundae
with whipped cream. Imagine eating
it very, very slowly, one delicious
bite at a time, your taste buds virtually
exploding with bliss.

Now, picture the buttons popping off the
waistband of your new $100 pants.

Girls in their
Summer Dresses
are *Beautiful*.

Girls in their
Summer Muumuus
are **not**.

date & **WEIGHT**	...... / ...... / ......
BREAKFAST	
LUNCH	
DINNER	
FRUIT N' VEG	① ② ③ ④ ⑤ ⑥ ⑦
WATER	① ② ③ ④ ⑤ ⑥ ⑦
hits & **BOMBS**	

date & **WEIGHT**	....../...... /	

BREAKFAST

LUNCH

DINNER

FRUIT N' VEG	① ② ③ ④ ⑤ ⑥ ⑦
WATER	① ② ③ ④ ⑤ ⑥ ⑦

hits & **BOMBS**

Samara Says

The only thing that stands between you and a slim waist is the **refrigerator.**

A COOKIE
IS A FLEETING PLEASURE.

THAT **GREAT** FEELING
YOU GET UPON SEEING A

THIN

YOU IN THE MIRROR
IS A LASTING PLEASURE.

date & **WEIGHT**	......./......./.......	

BREAKFAST

LUNCH

DINNER

FRUIT N' VEG	① ② ③ ④ ⑤ ⑥ ⑦
WATER	① ② ③ ④ ⑤ ⑥ ⑦

hits &
BOMBS

date & **WEIGHT**	......../......../............	
BREAKFAST		
LUNCH		
DINNER		
FRUIT N' VEG	① ② ③ ④ ⑤ ⑥ ⑦	
WATER	① ② ③ ④ ⑤ ⑥ ⑦	
hits & **BOMBS**		

THE BRITISH PHILOSOPHER,
GEORGE BERKELEY,
FAMOUSLY SAID,

"To <u>be</u> is to be perceived."

BUT FEW PEOPLE KNOW THAT
HE STOLE THIS LINE FROM HIS WIFE,
WHO ONCE ANNOUNCED,

"To be chubby, is to be perceived <u>chubby</u>."

THE REST IS HISTORY.

EXERCISE:
Before sitting down to dinner, close
your eyes and for one minute
visualize a pig slurping at the trough.

Kinda takes the edge off your appetite,
doesn't it?

date & **WEIGHT**	......../......../........	

BREAKFAST

LUNCH

DINNER

FRUIT N' VEG	① ② ③ ④ ⑤ ⑥ ⑦
WATER	① ② ③ ④ ⑤ ⑥ ⑦

hits & **BOMBS**

date & **WEIGHT**	...... / ...... /	
BREAKFAST		
LUNCH		
DINNER		
FRUIT N' VEG	① ② ③ ④ ⑤ ⑥ ⑦	
WATER	① ② ③ ④ ⑤ ⑥ ⑦	
hits & **BOMBS**		

18 C

IN THE 18TH CENTURY,
a *huge belly* was considered a sign
of wealth and good breeding.

IN THE 21ST CENTURY,
a *huge belly* is considered a sign
of poor eating habits and
bad breeding.

SO, HERE ARE YOUR CHOICES:
find a functioning time-travel machine
or *eat less.*

21C

The relationship between **FOOD INTAKE** and **WEIGHT GAIN** is a complicated science involving **CALORIES, COMPLEX CARBOHYDRATES,** and **ANIMAL PROTEINS**.

Let me simplify it for you:

FATS MAKE YOU FAT.

date & **WEIGHT**	....../....../......

BREAKFAST

LUNCH

DINNER

FRUIT N' VEG	① ② ③ ④ ⑤ ⑥ ⑦
WATER	① ② ③ ④ ⑤ ⑥ ⑦

hits &
BOMBS

date & **WEIGHT**	...... / ...... /	
BREAKFAST		
LUNCH		
DINNER		
FRUIT N' VEG	① ② ③ ④ ⑤ ⑥ ⑦	
WATER	① ② ③ ④ ⑤ ⑥ ⑦	
hits & **BOMBS**		

MENTAL EXERCISE:
pretend that donuts, cream cheese,
ice cream, and cake give you a *fatal disease.*

HELPFUL THOUGHT:
donuts, cream cheese, ice cream, and cake
can give you a fatal disease.

It's called **obesity.**

"They're called LOVE HANDLES "

because they are
something for your lover
to hold on to.

Come on,
hands are for holding, and fat folds
are for *losing*.

| date &
WEIGHT | ...... / ...... / ...... | |

BREAKFAST

LUNCH

DINNER

| **FRUIT N' VEG** | ① ② ③ ④ ⑤ ⑥ ⑦ |
| **WATER** | ① ② ③ ④ ⑤ ⑥ ⑦ |

hits &
BOMBS

date & **WEIGHT**	......./......./........	
BREAKFAST		
LUNCH		
DINNER		
FRUIT N' VEG	① ② ③ ④ ⑤ ⑥ ⑦	
WATER	① ② ③ ④ ⑤ ⑥ ⑦	
hits & **BOMBS**		

Samara Says

There is a reason the saying is not:
a **cupcake a day** keeps the doctor away.

One

of the great puzzlements:
what the heck does it mean
to **think thin?**

At last, an answer:
it means thinking with your mouth

closed.

date & **WEIGHT**	....../....../......	
BREAKFAST		
LUNCH		
DINNER		
FRUIT N' VEG	① ② ③ ④ ⑤ ⑥ ⑦	
WATER	① ② ③ ④ ⑤ ⑥ ⑦	
hits & **BOMBS**		

date & **WEIGHT**	......./......./.......	

BREAKFAST

LUNCH

DINNER

FRUIT N' VEG	① ② ③ ④ ⑤ ⑥ ⑦
WATER	① ② ③ ④ ⑤ ⑥ ⑦

hits & **BOMBS**

AS THE SAYING GOES,
"EXCESS IN MODERATION."
SO, CHOOSE YOUR EXCESS:

too much sex

too much money

too much to eat

EASY CHOICE, ISN'T IT?

"Dance, drink, and be merry."
Sound wrong to you?

THINK AGAIN.

date & **WEIGHT**	...... / ...... /	

BREAKFAST	

LUNCH	

DINNER	

FRUIT N' VEG	① ② ③ ④ ⑤ ⑥ ⑦
WATER	① ② ③ ④ ⑤ ⑥ ⑦

hits &
BOMBS

date & **WEIGHT**	......./......./.......	
BREAKFAST	
LUNCH	
DINNER	
FRUIT N' VEG	① ② ③ ④ ⑤ ⑥ ⑦
WATER	① ② ③ ④ ⑤ ⑥ ⑦
hits & **BOMBS**	

Before dinner,
stand naked
in front of the mirror
and examine your body, focusing in
on the problematic areas.

Now,
sit down at the dinner table.
That second helping doesn't look
as appetizing, does it?

WARNING: this exercise is bad for building self-esteem,
but good for breaking down fat.

PSYCHOLOGICAL FACT:

Eating is a substitute for kissing.
Kiss away!

date & **WEIGHT**	....../....../......	
BREAKFAST		
LUNCH		
DINNER		
FRUIT N' VEG	① ② ③ ④ ⑤ ⑥ ⑦	
WATER	① ② ③ ④ ⑤ ⑥ ⑦	
hits & **BOMBS**		

date & **WEIGHT**	....../....../......	
BREAKFAST		
LUNCH		
DINNER		
FRUIT N' VEG	① ② ③ ④ ⑤ ⑥ ⑦	
WATER	① ② ③ ④ ⑤ ⑥ ⑦	
hits & **BOMBS**		

Sure, inner beauty counts, but outer beauty counts **double**.

WE ALL KNOW HOW IMPORTANT IT IS TO LOVE YOURSELF.
But do you realize that if there is less of you to love, there's more self-love to go around?

date & **WEIGHT**	....../....../......	
BREAKFAST	
LUNCH	
DINNER	
FRUIT N' VEG	① ② ③ ④ ⑤ ⑥ ⑦
WATER	① ② ③ ④ ⑤ ⑥ ⑦
hits & **BOMBS**	

date & **WEIGHT**	...... / ...... /	
BREAKFAST	
LUNCH	
DINNER	
FRUIT N' VEG	① ② ③ ④ ⑤ ⑥ ⑦
WATER	① ② ③ ④ ⑤ ⑥ ⑦
hits & **BOMBS**	

Samara Says

A bit confusing but true: to have a French woman's body, you must **not eat** French bread, French toast, or French fries.

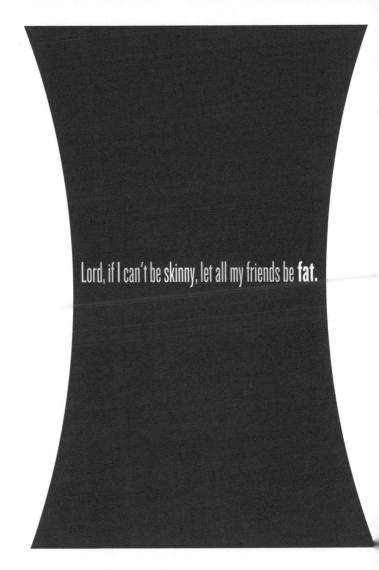

Lord, if I can't be skinny, let all my friends be **fat**.

date & **WEIGHT**	......../......../........

BREAKFAST

LUNCH

DINNER

FRUIT N' VEG	① ② ③ ④ ⑤ ⑥ ⑦
WATER	① ② ③ ④ ⑤ ⑥ ⑦

hits &
BOMBS

| date & **WEIGHT** | ....../....../...... | |

BREAKFAST

LUNCH

DINNER

| **FRUIT N' VEG** | ① ② ③ ④ ⑤ ⑥ ⑦ |
| **WATER** | ① ② ③ ④ ⑤ ⑥ ⑦ |

hits & **BOMBS**

Modern medical technology has provided us with all kinds of new options for losing weight such as having your jaw wired shut, or having your stomach surgically reduced in size, or taking high doses of amphetamines.

Of course, you can always use the old fashioned way and control your eating habits, but that's so passé.

THERE IS A REASON THAT JUSTICE IS PORTRAYED AS A WOMAN HOLDING A SCALE. IF YOU ARE TIPPING THAT SCALE, YOU ARE GUILTY.

date & **WEIGHT**	....../....../......	
BREAKFAST		
LUNCH		
DINNER		
FRUIT N' VEG	① ② ③ ④ ⑤ ⑥ ⑦	
WATER	① ② ③ ④ ⑤ ⑥ ⑦	
hits & **BOMBS**		

date & **WEIGHT**	...... / ...... /	
BREAKFAST		
LUNCH		
DINNER		
FRUIT N' VEG	① ② ③ ④ ⑤ ⑥ ⑦	
WATER	① ② ③ ④ ⑤ ⑥ ⑦	
hits & **BOMBS**		

Sara Lee,
Betty Crocker,
Aunt Jemima…

They sound like
nice women,
but they're really

evil.

ON

those instant-makeover reality TV shows,
contestants get
tummy tucks, liposuction, and Brazilian butt-lifts.

Exercise:
imagine that you are on your own,
personal episode of

"Slow Motion Makeover."

No scalpels allowed.

date & **WEIGHT**	........./........./.........	
BREAKFAST		
LUNCH		
DINNER		
FRUIT N' VEG	① ② ③ ④ ⑤ ⑥ ⑦	
WATER	① ② ③ ④ ⑤ ⑥ ⑦	
hits & **BOMBS**		

date & **WEIGHT**	......../......../........	
BREAKFAST		
LUNCH		
DINNER		
FRUIT N' VEG	① ② ③ ④ ⑤ ⑥ ⑦	
WATER	① ② ③ ④ ⑤ ⑥ ⑦	
hits & **BOMBS**		

Samara Says

Dedicating yourself to developing a slim, attractive body is a such a superficial pursuit. **Let's hear it for superficiality!**

A new report from the
AMERICAN MEDICAL ASSOCIATION
states that a clear sign of an over-eating
disorder is increased body weight.

Smart, those docs, aren't they?

date & **WEIGHT**	...... / ...... / ......
BREAKFAST	
LUNCH	
DINNER	
FRUIT N' VEG	① ② ③ ④ ⑤ ⑥ ⑦
WATER	① ② ③ ④ ⑤ ⑥ ⑦
hits & **BOMBS**	

date & **WEIGHT**	...... / ...... /	
BREAKFAST	
LUNCH	
DINNER	
FRUIT N' VEG	① ② ③ ④ ⑤ ⑥ ⑦
WATER	① ② ③ ④ ⑤ ⑥ ⑦
hits & **BOMBS**	

Just **DON'T** eat it!

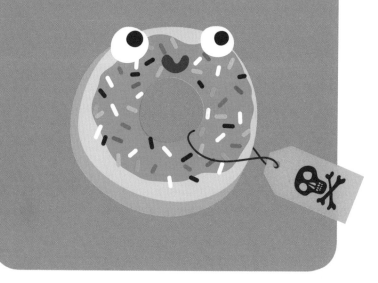

Overweight women often
ask skinny women,

"What's your secret?"

Well, I hate to break it to you, but
the secret is: **EAT LESS!**

Big friggin' secret.

date & **WEIGHT**	......./......./.......	

BREAKFAST

LUNCH

DINNER

FRUIT N' VEG	① ② ③ ④ ⑤ ⑥ ⑦
WATER	① ② ③ ④ ⑤ ⑥ ⑦

hits &
BOMBS

date & **WEIGHT**	...... / ...... /	
BREAKFAST	
LUNCH	
DINNER	
FRUIT N' VEG	① ② ③ ④ ⑤ ⑥ ⑦
WATER	① ② ③ ④ ⑤ ⑥ ⑦
hits & **BOMBS**	

You know you are
thinking about food too much
when during *sex*
you call out the
name of a condiment.

You know those
"friends"
who say,
"You don't need to go on a diet!"
when you refrain from
taking a slice of pie a la mode?

Well, they aren't really
your friends—
they want you to be
fat
like them.

date & **WEIGHT**	...... / ...... / ......
BREAKFAST	
LUNCH	
DINNER	
FRUIT N' VEG	① ② ③ ④ ⑤ ⑥ ⑦
WATER	① ② ③ ④ ⑤ ⑥ ⑦
hits & **BOMBS**	

date & **WEIGHT**	.... / .... /	

BREAKFAST

LUNCH

DINNER

FRUIT N' VEG	① ② ③ ④ ⑤ ⑥ ⑦
WATER	① ② ③ ④ ⑤ ⑥ ⑦

hits &
BOMBS

Gluttony
is one of the seven
deadly sins.

IT'S BAD ENOUGH BEING FAT,
BUT TO BE A SINNER ON TOP OF IT?

THAT REALLY DOESN'T MAKE A BAG OF CHIPS
WORTH IT

Food licked off cooking utensils has no calories. We're talking cookie dough on a spatula or whipped cream on a whisk.

This has not been proven yet; our lab staff is still working on it—meanwhile, they've gained 47 pounds.

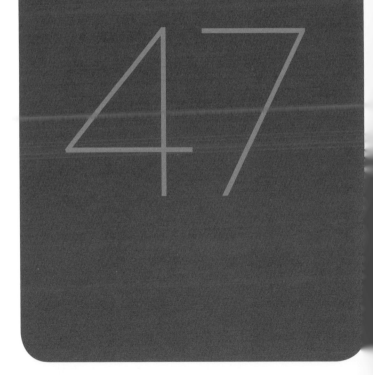

date & **WEIGHT**	.... / .... / ....

BREAKFAST

LUNCH

DINNER

FRUIT N' VEG	① ② ③ ④ ⑤ ⑥ ⑦
WATER	① ② ③ ④ ⑤ ⑥ ⑦

hits &
BOMBS

date & **WEIGHT**	........../........../..............

BREAKFAST	
LUNCH	
DINNER	
FRUIT N' VEG	① ② ③ ④ ⑤ ⑥ ⑦
WATER	① ② ③ ④ ⑤ ⑥ ⑦
hits & **BOMBS**	

Italian Mouth Options:

STUFF IT WITH
Pizza

STUFF IT WITH
Lasagna

STUFF IT WITH
Tiramisu

PUCKER IT UP AND
KISS A HANDSOME
ITALIAN MAN
FULL ON HIS
DELICIOUS LIPS!

NOTE: ONLY ONE OF THE ABOVE IS AVAILABLE TO EACH CUSTOMER.

REMEMBER THAT OLD RHYME, "CANDY IS DANDY, BUT LIQUOR IS QUICKER"? WELL HERE'S THE MISSING THIRD LINE: "AND BOTH MAKE YOU THICKER."

date & **WEIGHT**	...... / ...... /	

BREAKFAST	

LUNCH	

DINNER	

FRUIT N' VEG	① ② ③ ④ ⑤ ⑥ ⑦
WATER	① ② ③ ④ ⑤ ⑥ ⑦

hits & **BOMBS**	

date & **WEIGHT**	....../....../......
BREAKFAST	
LUNCH	
DINNER	
FRUIT N' VEG	① ② ③ ④ ⑤ ⑥ ⑦
WATER	① ② ③ ④ ⑤ ⑥ ⑦
hits & **BOMBS**	

Samara Says

If dieting takes courage, then
Eating is For Sissies!
Now aren't you ashamed?

WHEN TOLD THAT
PEOPLE WERE HUNGRY WITH
NO BREAD TO EAT, MARIE ANTOINETTE
FAMOUSLY SAID,

"LET THEM EAT CAKE!"

✠

HISTORIANS NOW AGREE THAT
MS. ANTOINETTE WAS A
HORRIBLY VAIN WOMAN WHO WANTED
EVERYONE ELSE TO BE HEAVIER
THAN SHE WAS.
A KINDER, GENTLER MARIE ANTOINETTE
WOULD HAVE SAID,

"LET THEM EAT HIGH FIBER CRACKERS!"

date & **WEIGHT**	......../......../........	

BREAKFAST

LUNCH

DINNER

FRUIT N' VEG ① ② ③ ④ ⑤ ⑥ ⑦

WATER ① ② ③ ④ ⑤ ⑥ ⑦

hits & **BOMBS**

date & **WEIGHT**	.... / .... / ....
BREAKFAST	
LUNCH	
DINNER	
FRUIT N' VEG	① ② ③ ④ ⑤ ⑥ ⑦
WATER	① ② ③ ④ ⑤ ⑥ ⑦
hits & **BOMBS**	

THERE ARE **TWO** WAYS TO CALCULATE
YOUR BODY MASS INDEX:

1. Take your weight in pounds and divide by
the square of your height in inches, then
multiply the result by 703. If your BMI is over
25 you are overweight; over 30, obese.

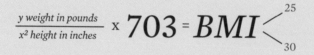

$$\frac{y \text{ weight in pounds}}{x^2 \text{ height in inches}} \times 703 = BMI \begin{cases} 25 \\ 30 \end{cases}$$

2. Strip in front of the mirror and take a cold,
hard look. Either way, you know what to do next.

date & **WEIGHT**	...... / ...... /	

BREAKFAST

LUNCH

DINNER

FRUIT N' VEG	① ② ③ ④ ⑤ ⑥ ⑦
WATER	① ② ③ ④ ⑤ ⑥ ⑦

hits &
BOMBS

You *are* what you eat.

For example if you eat a pork chop . . .

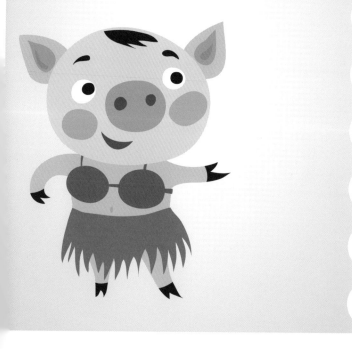

When you are
walking down the street,

look at a woman who is fatter than you are.

Feeling better about yourself?

Good.

That was for your self-esteem.

Later on, look at a woman who is thinner than you are.

Feeling badly about yourself?

Good.

That was for your motivation.

date & **WEIGHT**	......./......./.......	
BREAKFAST		
LUNCH		
DINNER		
FRUIT N' VEG	① ② ③ ④ ⑤ ⑥ ⑦	
WATER	① ② ③ ④ ⑤ ⑥ ⑦	

hits &
BOMBS

Do you see that fat blond woman?

Do you actually think that she's having more fun?

No, blondes don't have more fun—thin women do.

date & **WEIGHT**	......./......./.......	
BREAKFAST		
LUNCH		
DINNER		
FRUIT N' VEG	① ② ③ ④ ⑤ ⑥ ⑦	
WATER	① ② ③ ④ ⑤ ⑥ ⑦	
hits & **BOMBS**		

ɗate & **WEIGHT**	......./......./............

BREAKFAST	
LUNCH	
DINNER	
FRUIT N' VEG	① ② ③ ④ ⑤ ⑥ ⑦
WATER	① ② ③ ④ ⑤ ⑥ ⑦
ɦits & **BOMBS**	

EXERCISE: Buy a copy of *Vogue*.
Look at the models and say out loud.

"They look ridiculous!
They look sickly!
They look awful."

Now, be honest with yourself—
don't those words sound *hollow*?

Remember when you could happily take a nude swim with your beau?

It was called "skinny dipping" for a reason.

date & WEIGHT	....../......	

BREAKFAST	

LUNCH	

DINNER	

FRUIT N' VEG	① ② ③ ④ ⑤ ⑥ ⑦
WATER	① ② ③ ④ ⑤ ⑥ ⑦

hits &
BOMBS

date & **WEIGHT**	......../......../................
BREAKFAST	
LUNCH	
DINNER	
FRUIT N' VEG	① ② ③ ④ ⑤ ⑥ ⑦
WATER	① ② ③ ④ ⑤ ⑥ ⑦
hits & **BOMBS**	

When
THE BIBLE SAYS,
"GOD HELPS
THOSE
WHO HELP
THEMSELVES,"
IT IS **Not**
REFERRING TO
SECOND
HELPINGS.

Let's be naughty.

Break the rules. Be devilish.
That's right—put jam on your toast. . .

Okay, that's enough.

*d*ate &**WEIGHT**	...../...../.....	
BREAKFAST		
LUNCH		
DINNER		
FRUIT N' VEG	① ② ③ ④ ⑤ ⑥ ⑦	
WATER	① ② ③ ④ ⑤ ⑥ ⑦	
*h*its &**BOMBS**		

date & **WEIGHT**	......./......./.......	
BREAKFAST		
LUNCH		
DINNER		
FRUIT N' VEG	① ② ③ ④ ⑤ ⑥ ⑦	
WATER	① ② ③ ④ ⑤ ⑥ ⑦	
hits & **BOMBS**		

"Full mind and spirit.
Empty stomach."

REMEMBER THE OLD EXCUSE:
"I just come from a family with big bones"?
Right, that's what the dinosaurs said.

date & **WEIGHT**	...... / ...... /	
BREAKFAST		
LUNCH		
DINNER		
FRUIT N' VEG	① ② ③ ④ ⑤ ⑥ ⑦	
WATER	① ② ③ ④ ⑤ ⑥ ⑦	

hits &
BOMBS

date & **WEIGHT**	....../....../......	

BREAKFAST

LUNCH

DINNER

FRUIT N' VEG	① ② ③ ④ ⑤ ⑥ ⑦
WATER	① ② ③ ④ ⑤ ⑥ ⑦

hits & **BOMBS**

Have you ever seen those people who wear pins that say,

"LOSE WEIGHT NOW, ASK ME HOW."

Well, here is what they'll tell you in two hours, in two words,

"EAT LESS!"

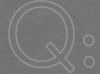

QUIZ QUESTION:
What's the difference between
eating between meals
and **eating five meals a day?**

Whatever the difference,
it's not one your
bathroom scale makes.

date & **WEIGHT**	...... / ...... /	
BREAKFAST		
LUNCH		
DINNER		
FRUIT N' VEG	① ② ③ ④ ⑤ ⑥ ⑦	
WATER	① ② ③ ④ ⑤ ⑥ ⑦	
hits & **BOMBS**		

date & **WEIGHT**	...... / ...... / ......
BREAKFAST	
LUNCH	
DINNER	
FRUIT N' VEG	① ② ③ ④ ⑤ ⑥ ⑦
WATER	① ② ③ ④ ⑤ ⑥ ⑦
hits & **BOMBS**	

Oysters on the half shell,
asparagus, and strawberries
are all aphrodisiacs.

Have an aphrodisiac meal and
then burn it off in bed.

(Wink, wink)

LET'S BE PERFECTLY CLEAR:
that awful emptiness you feel in your stomach
after one day without food is called **hunger,**
but that capricious appetite you feel in
your stomach between lunch and dinner
is called **indulgence.**

date & **WEIGHT**	......./......./.......	

BREAKFAST

LUNCH

DINNER

FRUIT N' VEG	① ② ③ ④ ⑤ ⑥ ⑦
WATER	① ② ③ ④ ⑤ ⑥ ⑦

hits &
BOMBS

date & **WEIGHT**	...... / ...... /	
BREAKFAST		
LUNCH		
DINNER		
FRUIT N' VEG	① ② ③ ④ ⑤ ⑥ ⑦	
WATER	① ② ③ ④ ⑤ ⑥ ⑦	
hits & **BOMBS**		